Table of Contents

Introduction

Lyme disease is an infectious disease caused by the bacteria Borrelia burgdorferi. B. burgdorferi is transmitted to humans by a bite from an infected black-legged or deer tick. The tick becomes infected after feeding on infected deer, birds, or mice.

The lyme diet is great if you want to take down inflammation in your body and boost your immune system!

By the end of this journey you will be very healthy. Basically, a huge part of fighting this disease is having a proper diet. Killing off the Lyme from the inside with antibiotics is one step, but it's important to starve the disease of foods that fuel it. You must not give the bacteria anything which would feed it or give it more power or strength. It's also really important to remove foods from the diet which are inflammatory, as this can cause added trouble and pain. And with that, this brings me to the Lyme diet!

This book contains varieties of healthy and anti-inflammatory diets that will help treat and prevent against Lyme disease.

Healthy Lyme disease recipes

Carrot Almond Pancakes

These carrot almond pancakes may look a little different than what you're used to, but they taste sweet, nutty and are very satisfying. Top the pancakes with a teaspoon of raw honey and some blueberries for a complete breakfast treat. Have this unique gluten-free pancake recipe for your next breakfast!

Serves: 3

Ingredients

- 1 cup peeled and grated carrots (2-3 carrots)

- ¼ cup almonds

- 1 slice fresh ginger (1/8-inch thick)

- 1 teaspoon ground flaxseed

- 2 tablespoons unsweetened shredded coconut

- ½ teaspoon ground cinnamon

- 1 egg

- ¼ teaspoon sea salt

- ½ teaspoon vanilla

- 1-2 tablespoons Ghee

- 1 teaspoon raw honey

- Blueberries (optional)

Instructions

1. Place the grated carrots in a medium-sized bowl.

2. Place the almonds, ginger and flaxseed in the bowl of a food processor. Pulse 5-6 times until the almonds are finely ground.

3. Add the almond mixture and all of the remaining ingredients, except for the ghee, honey and blueberries, to the grated carrots.

4. Heat the ghee in a small frying pan over medium heat for 2 minutes, or until hot.

5. Pour two ¼-cup portions of pancake batter into the frying pan, and cook for about 3 minutes per side, or until lightly browned.

6. Repeat with the remaining batter.

7. Top with honey and blueberries if desired, and serve hot.

Slow Cooked Brown Rice Risotto and Mushrooms

Don't have time stir that risotto? No problem with this recipe for Brown Rice Risotto and Mushrooms. Let the slow cooker do all the work.

Serves: 4

Ingredients

- 3 tablespoons extra virgin olive oil, divided

- 2 shallots, peeled and chopped

- 2 cloves garlic, peeled and chopped

- ¾ cup short grain brown rice

- 8 oz. baby bella or crimini mushrooms, sliced

- 2½ cups vegetable broth

- 1 teaspoon salt

- 2 tablespoons each, freshly chopped parsley and basil

- ½ teaspoon each, freshly chopped thyme and mint

- 1 teaspoon, freshly chopped dill

Instructions

1. Heat the oil in a large fry page over medium-
    high heat for 1 minute or until hot.

2. Add the shallots and saute for one minute.
    Stir in the garlic and cook 30 seconds.

3. Add the remaining oil and uncooked rice and
    cook stirring for about 2 minutes.

4. Add the mushrooms and fry for 3 minutes or
    until just limp. Stir in salt.

5. Add the fried ingredients to the slow cooker.

6. Add the vegetable broth and stir well.

7. Cover and cook on low for 2 hours. Stir in
    the herbs in the last ½ hour.

8. Serve immediately.

Moroccan Spice-Rubbed Salmon

You may have never used the spices in this recipe for Moroccan Spice-Rubbed Salmon, but don't hesitate to give this recipe a try. It might just open a whole new world of delicious possibilities to you and your family.

Serves: 2

Ingredients

Rub

- 1 teaspoon garlic powder
- ½ teaspoon onion powder
- ½ teaspoon ground turmeric
- ¼ teaspoon sea salt

- ¼ teaspoon dried oregano

- ½ teaspoon garam masala or curry powder

- 1/8 teaspoon ground ginger

Fish

- 2 (6-ounce) salmon filets

- Topping (not pictured)

- 1 small onion, sliced in rounds

- 1 tablespoon extra virgin olive oil

Instructions

1. Preheat the oven to 450°F.

2. Combine all the ingredients for the rub.

3. Spread the rub on the flesh side of the salmon filets.

4. Cook the fish without turning for 8 minutes,
    or until the fish flakes easily with a fork.

5. While the fish is cooking, sauté the onion in
    the oil.

6. Place the fried onion rounds on top of the
    fish for the last 2 minutes of cooking.

Cauliflower Carrot Soup

This smooth soup combines two basic vegetables
into a delicious medley of flavors. Serve with the
Savory Vegetable and Herb Biscotti.

Serves: 4

Ingredients

- 2 tablespoons extra virgin olive oil

- 1 medium onion, chopped

- 2 cloves garlic, chopped

- ½ small head cauliflower (about 8 ounces) cut into florets

- 2 carrots peeled and chopped

- 1 quart Vegetable Stock (page 235)

- 2 tablespoon chopped parsley

- 1 tablespoon chopped chives

- 1 teaspoon chopped rosemary

- 1 teaspoon freshly chopped dill

- 1 teaspoon celery salt

- ½ teaspoon salt

- 1 ½ cup coconut milk

Instructions

1. Heat the oil in a 2-quart sauce pot over medium-high heat for 1 minute or until hot.

2. Fry the onions for 3 minutes or until limp.

3. Add the garlic, cauliflower and carrots and saute for 5 minutes.

4. Add the remaining ingredients and stir well to combine.

5. Bring the soup to a boil over medium-high heat. Lower the heat to medium and simmer for 35 minutes.

6. Pour the soup into a blender container. Cover the container. Remove the center cup from the cover.

7. Place a clean, folded kitchen towel over the blender cover and press down with your hand.

8. Puree the soup until smooth.

9. Serve immediately and refrigerate leftovers.

Nutty Coconut Delight

This recipe is a real treat. You are urged to keep your intake of sweets to a minimum, so restrict yourself to one. However, once you taste these treats, stopping at one might be easier said than done!

Serves: 15

Ingredients

- ¼ cup Ghee

- ½ cup raw honey

- ½ cup almonds

- 1 teaspoon cinnamon

- ¾ cup unsweetened coconut

- ½ cup walnuts, chopped

Instructions

1. Preheat the oven to 350°F.

2. Place the ghee, honey, almonds and cinnamon in the bowl of a food processor fitted with a steel blade. Pulse 6 or 7 times, or until the nuts are ground.

3. Grease the bottom of an 8-inch square baking pan. Spread the nut and honey mixture over the bottom of the greased pan.

4. Sprinkle the coconut over the honey nut mixture, and then sprinkle the chopped walnuts over the coconut.

5. Place the pan in the oven and bake for 15-20 minutes, or until the edges bubble and begin to brown.

6. Allow the pan to cool and then refrigerate it for several hours or overnight.

7. Scoop the mixture into balls using a small ice cream scoop or serving spoon.

8. Serve immediately and refrigerate any leftovers.

Chocolate Coconut Macaroons

You'll have a hard time believing that these spectacular treats are gluten-free, dairy-free, egg-free, vegan and don't require any cooking –

making them a raw food delight. What more can you ask for?

Serves: 10

Ingredients

- 2 tablespoons cocoa powder, unsweetened

- ¼ cup extra virgin coconut oil, softened

- 1 teaspoon pure vanilla extract

- 2 tablespoons maple syrup or coconut palm nectar

- Pinch of salt

- ¾ cup unsweetened shredded coconut

- ⅔ cup very finely chopped pecans, or nut of your choice

Instructions

1. Combine the cocoa, coconut oil, vanilla, syrup and salt.

2. Stir well to combine completely. The mixture will have the appearance of melted chocolate.

3. Add the coconut and stir with a spoon until it's well incorporated into the chocolate mixture.

4. Line a cookie sheet with parchment paper.

5. Scoop the mixture into balls using a small ice cream scoop or serving spoon.

6. Place the chopped nuts on a flat plate. Roll each ball in the nuts until well coated.

7. Place each macaroon on the parchment lined tray and refrigerate.

8. Once chilled, about 30 minutes, the treats are ready to eat.

Herb Scrambled Eggs with Shitake Mushrooms

This recipe for Herb Scrambled Eggs with Shitake Mushrooms can top the Brown Rice Pancakes or be eaten alone. When served on the Brown Rice Pancake it makes a wonderful meal that you can serve guests for brunch.

Serves: 2

Ingredients

- 1 teaspoon extra virgin olive oil

- 1 cup chopped shitake mushrooms

- 2 scallions, white part only, chopped

- 1 small clove of garlic, chopped

- 2 teaspoons of freshly chopped herbs, such as parsley, oregano, tarragon or lemon thyme

- ½ teaspoon salt

- 2 eggs beaten

Instructions

1. Heat the oil over medium heat in a fry pan for 1 minute.

2. Add the scallions, garlic and mushrooms and cook for two minutes.

3. Combine the herbs and eggs and mix well with a fork.

4. Pour the eggs into a fry pan and cook for two minutes mixing with a fork to scramble.

5. Serve on Brown Rice Pancake.

Apricot Oat Muffins

Try this muffin for breakfast or a mid-morning snack with a cup of ginger tea. It's sweet, fruity and nutty and a nice change of pace for Phase 2.

Serves: 6

Ingredients

- ⅔ cup (62 grams) quick oats

- 1 tablespoon chia seeds or 1 egg (if using egg, reduce the brown rice milk by ¼ cup)

- 1 cup Brown Rice Milk

- 1 teaspoon vanilla

- ¼ cup maple syrup

- ¼ safflower oil

- ¾ cup (100 grams) brown rice flour

- ¼ teaspoon salt

- ½ teaspoon cinnamon

- ¼ teaspoon ground ginger

- 2 teaspoons Homemade Baking Powder

- ⅓ cup finely chopped dried apricot

Topping

- 2 tablespoons quick oats

- 3 tablespoons chopped pecans

- ¼ teaspoon cinnamon

Instructions

1. Preheat the oven to 350°F.

2. Grease a 6-cup muffin pan and set aside.

3. Combine the oats, chia seeds or egg, rice milk, vanilla, maple syrup and oil.

4. Stir well and allow to stand while the oven is preheating.

5. Combine the flour, salt, cinnamon, ginger and baking powder in small bowl.

6. Add the flour mixture into the oatmeal mixture and stir well. Stir in chopped apricots.

7. Fill each muffin cup with a scant ⅓ cup of batter.

8. Combine the topping ingredients and sprinkle the mixture over the muffins.

9. Bake in the preheated oven for 25 minutes, or until a toothpick inserted into the middle of the muffin comes out clean.

10. Allow the muffins to cool in the pan completely before removing. Refrigerate or freeze leftovers.

Stir-Fried Brown Rice and Vegetables

Brown rice has a nutty taste, and stir-frying gives it a little crunch and enhances the flavor. Adding chopped nuts and blueberries ties all the flavors together, making this recipe for Stir-Fried Brown Rice and Vegetables a satisfying, meatless meal.

Serves: 2

Ingredients

- 3 tablespoons extra virgin olive oil, divided
- 4 scallions, chopped
- 2 cloves garlic, chopped
- 1 cup broccoli, broken into small florets or coarsely chopped
- 1 cup shredded carrots
- 1 cup sliced celery
- 1 cup cooked brown rice
- ½ teaspoon extra virgin olive oil

- 1 egg, lightly beaten

- 2 tablespoons chopped, toasted almonds or walnuts

- 2 tablespoons blueberries

Instructions

1. Heat 2 tablespoons of the oil in a large frying pan over medium-high heat for about 2 minutes, or until hot.

2. Add the scallions, garlic, broccoli, carrots and celery and stir fry for 3 minutes, or until nicely browned.

3. Add the remaining 1 tablespoon of oil and the rice, and stir fry for another minute.

4. Remove the rice and vegetables from the frying pan.

5. Add the ½ teaspoon of oil to the frying pan and heat for 30 seconds.

6. Pour the egg into the frying pan, making sure to cover the bottom of the pan.

7. Cook for 1 minute, turn, and cook for 1 minute, or until set. Remove the egg and slice into thin strips.

8. Top the rice with the egg strips, and add the chopped nuts and apricots or blueberries. Serve immediately.

Brown and Wild Rice Cauliflower and Mushroom Curry

This recipe uses all leftovers so you can be eating dinner in just a matter of minutes.

Serves: 4

Ingredients

- 2 tablespoons coconut oil or extra virgin olive oil

- 1 small onion, chopped

- 1 clove garlic, chopped

- 4 oz. mushrooms, sliced

- 1½ cups cooked brown and wild rice

- 6 oz. cooked, steamed cauliflower

- 1½ cups baby spinach leaves

- 1 teaspoon curry powder

- ½ teaspoon tumeric

- ¼ teaspoon cumin

- 1 teaspoon sea salt

- ½ teaspoon celery salt

- ½ teaspoon garlic powder

- 1 tablespoon each, chopped parsley and chopped basil

- 1 cup coconut milk

- ½ cup vegetable stock

- 2 tablespoons chopped walnuts

- 2 tablespoons unsweetened coconut

Instructions

1. Heat the coconut oil in a large fry pan over medium-high heat for 1 minute.

2. Add the onions and fry for two minutes or until limp.

3. Add the garlic and fry for 30 seconds.

4. Add the mushrooms and fry for three minutes or until limp.

5. Add the rice and the remaining ingredients except the spinach, chopped walnuts and shredded coconut. Stir well and cook for 2 minutes.

6. Stir in the spinach and cook for 1 minute, just to warm the spinach. Do not allow it to wilt.

7. Serve topped with chopped walnuts and shredded coconut.

Deviled Eggs or Egg Salad

This old-time favorite has made a recent comeback. So, if you haven't had it in a while, why not give it a try?

Serves: 12

Ingredients

- 6 eggs, hard boiled and peeled

- 3 tablespoons Herb Mayonnaise (page 271)

- 1 tablespoon mustard

- ¼ teaspoon sea salt

Instructions

1. Cut the peeled, cooked eggs in half lengthwise. R

2. emove the yolks to a small bowl and add the remaining ingredients.

3. Break the yolks up with a fork and continue to mash until the mixture is smooth.

4. Spoon the filling back into the egg whites, or, if desired, pipe it back into the whites using a pastry bag fitted with a star tip.

Pickled Beets

Pickled beets are great as an addition to a salad, or as a stand-alone side dish served hot or cold.

Serves: 4-6

Ingredients

- 1 bunch (4-5) beets (about 2 pounds worth)

- ¼ cup cider vinegar

- ½ cup water

- 1 small onion, sliced

- 1 clove garlic, peeled and thinly sliced

- ½ teaspoon sea salt

- 2 tablespoons raw honey

Instructions

1. Place the beets in a quart saucepan and cover them with water.

2. Cover the pan, and bring to a boil over high heat. Lower the heat to medium-high and cook for 45-50 minutes, or until a knife inserted in the middle of a beet comes out easily.

3. Drain, cool and peel the beets, and then slice them into ¼-inch thick slices.

4. Return the sliced beets to the saucepan and add the vinegar, water, onion, garlic and salt.

5. Cook over high heat until the mixture comes to a boil. Lower the heat and cook for about 10 minutes, or until tender.

6. Remove the beets from the heat and allow them to cool. Stir in the honey.

7. Serve hot or cold.

Poached Eggs Florentine With Béarnaise Sauce

This recipe is perfect if you are hosting brunch, or if you enjoy a fancy breakfast at home.

Serves: 4

Ingredients

- 1 recipe Béarnaise Sauce

- 1 tablespoon Ghee (page 254) or extra virgin olive oil

- 1 small shallot, minced

- 1 small clove garlic, crushed

- 1 bag (1 pound) baby spinach

- 3 cups water

- 4 eggs

- 1 teaspoon raw apple cider vinegar

- Chopped parsley **(optional)**

Instructions

1. Prepare the Béarnaise Sauce and set aside.

2. Heat the ghee or oil in a small frying pan.

3. Add the shallot and garlic and fry over medium heat for 2 minutes, or until limp.

4. Add the spinach and fry for 2 minutes, or until just limp. Set aside.

5. Pour the water into a frying pan, and bring it to a boil.

6. Crack each egg into a separate custard cup.

7. Once the water boils, add the vinegar and stir vigorously until a whirlpool forms.

8. Add the eggs one at a time, and poach for about 2 minutes. Spoon any floating

9. egg white back over the poaching egg.
Continue until all the eggs are poached.

10. If necessary, reheat the spinach for a
minute.

11. Divide the spinach and place on four plates.

12. Top each portion of spinach with a poached
egg, and spoon Béarnaise Sauce over each.

13. Garnish with chopped parsley if desired.

Olive Tapenade Baked Haddock

Top this mild white fish with green olives for a maximum burst of flavor.

Ingredients

- 1 lb. skinless haddock fillet, cut in four pieces
- ½ teaspoon each, salt and garlic powder
- 1 teaspoon mustard or ½ teaspoon mustard powder
- 2 teaspoons extra virgin olive oil
- 16 large pitted green olives
- ½ teaspoon freshly chopped oregano
- ½ teaspoon freshly chopped lemon thyme

Instructions

1. Preheat the oven to 425°.

2. Place the fish on a baking dish and sprinkle with salt, garlic powder and mustard powder.

3. Drizzle olive oil over each fillet.

4. Place the olives and herbs in the bowl of a food processor fitted with a steel blade.

5. Pulse 5 or 6 times until evenly chopped.

6. Spread the chopped olives evenly over the fish fillets.

7. Bake for 18-20 minutes or until fish flakes easily with a fork.

Steamed Vegetables and Brown and Wild Rice with Fresh Herb Vinaigrette

Leftover rice and vegetables make a great salad when topped with our homemade Fresh Herb Vinaigrette.

Serves: 4

Ingredients

- 2 cups cooked brown and wild rice

- 3 ounces steamed green beans

- 1 cup steamed bok choy

- 1 cup steamed julienned carrots

- 1 recipe of Fresh Herb Vinaigrette

Instructions

1. Place the cooked rice on a serving plate and top with the green beans, bok choy and carrots.

2. Spoon a small amount of the vinaigrette over the vegetables, and serve the remaining vinaigrette on the side.

Shredded Carrot Salad

Make this Shredded Carrot Salad to take to work for lunch, or serve as a dinner side dish with Almond and Herb Crusted Tilapia

Serves: 4

Ingredients

- 2 cups shredded carrots (about 8 ounces)
- ¼ cup Homemade Mayonnaise
- 1½ teaspoons raw honey
- 1 teaspoon freshly chopped chives
- ½ teaspoon lemon thyme
- 2 teaspoons raw apple cider vinegar
- 2 tablespoons chopped walnuts

Instructions

1. Combine all the ingredients in a bowl and stir well.

2. Refrigerate for at least an hour before serving.

Béarnaise Sauce

This sauce is delicious on poached eggs, but can also be a welcome addition that will add a little spark to steamed vegetables or broiled fish.

Serves: ¾ cup

Ingredients

- 2 egg yolks

- 1 teaspoon chopped tarragon or lemon thyme

- ½ tablespoon raw apple cider vinegar

- 1/3 cup Ghee

Instructions

1. Place all the ingredients, except for the ghee, in a blender container and blend on High for 30 seconds.

2. With the blender running, slowly drizzle the ghee into the container until it forms an emulsion.

3. Remove the sauce from the container and use immediately, or refrigerate until ready to use.

Savory Vegetable and Herb Biscotti

These savory biscuits are an excellent accompaniment to have with a soup or salad. Break one up into pieces and use them atop a salad like a crouton.

Serves: 10

Ingredients

- 1½ cups almond flour

- 2 tablespoons flaxseed meal

- ¼ cup fresh spinach, chopped

- 1 tablespoon onions, chopped

- ¼ cup carrots, chopped

- ¼ teaspoon celery salt

- 1 teaspoon salt

- 1 teaspoon garlic powder

- 1 teaspoon dried basil

- 1 teaspoon Herbes de Provence

- 2 tablespoons extra virgin olive oil

Instructions

1. Preheat the oven to 375°F.

2. Place all the ingredients in the bowl of a food processor. Pulse on and off about 10 times or until the mixture begins to form a bowl.

3. Line a small baking sheet with parchment paper.

4. Remove the mixture and place it on the parchment paper. Form the mixture into a 7 x 3½ x ¾-inch loaf.

5. Bake in the preheated oven for 30-35 minutes or until the edges start to brown.

6. Cool on a rack for 30 minutes.

7. Cut the cooled loaf into 10 half-inch diagonal slices on a cutting board with a serrated edge knife.

8. Put the slices flat side down onto the parchment lined sheet.

9. Place the sheet back in the oven and bake 12-15 minutes, turning mid-way, until the Biscotti is lightly browned. Do not over bake or else they will taste burned.

Berry Frozen Dessert

This newly developed Berry Frozen Dessert recipe
is a delicious new dessert for Lyme Inflammation.

Serves: 4

Ingredients

- 6 oz. frozen strawberries, raspberries, blackberries or blueberries or a combination
- 1 cup coconut milk, canned
- a pinch of sea salt
- 1 teaspoon vanilla
- 2-4 drops stevia, optional

Instructions

1. Put the frozen berries into the food processor. Pulse several times until coarsely chopped.

2. Add the remaining ingredients. Pulse until smooth.

3. Place in a container and freeze for two hours before serving.

Homemade Brown Rice Milk

Serves: 2 cups

Ingredients

- ½ cup brown rice

- 4 cups filtered water, divided

Instructions

1. Soak the brown rice overnight in two cups of water.

2. Drain the rice and place in a blender container and add 2 cups of new water.

3. Blend for about 2 minutes. The rice will be pulverized and settle at the bottom of the blender container.

4. Line a colander or a sieve with cheesecloth. Pour the liquid into the cheesecloth to strain out the milk.

5. Squeeze out all the of the liquid from the mixture into the bowl.

6. Disregard the rice pulp.

7. Store the rice milk in a sealed container in the refrigerator for up to two days or freeze the excess.

Almond and Herb Crusted Tilapia

The coating in this recipe, which replaces breadcrumbs, is one of many that you will find in the various Phases of this book. Best of all, these replacements add variety to your menus.

Serves: 4

Ingredients

- ⅔ cup amond meal
- 2 teaspoons each freshly chopped parsley, thyme, oregano and chives
- 1 clove garlic, crushed
- ½ teaspoon sea salt
- 4 (4- to 6-ounce) tilapia filets

- 3 tablespoons coconut oil or Ghee

- Herb Mayonnaise

Instructions

1. Combine the almond meal, herbs, garlic and salt on a dinner plate. Mix well.

2. Coat both sides of each filet with the mixture. Press the crumbs into the fish using your hands.

3. Place the fish on a small rack and let it sit in the refrigerator, uncovered, for at least 30 minutes, to allow the crumbs to dry and set in place.

4. Heat the oil or ghee in a frying pan over medium-high heat for about 3 minutes, or until hot.

5. Place the fish in the pan and cook for 5-7 minutes per side (depending on the thickness of the fish), until the crust is nicely browned.

6. Serve immediately, with Herb Mayonnaise.

Pumpkin Cranberry Muffins

These delicious Pumpkin Cranberry Muffins make a wonderful breakfast or dinnertime accompaniment.

Serves: 6

Ingredients

- ¾ cup canned, or cooked and pureed, pumpkin
- ¼ cup Cran-Raspberry Sauce
- 3 tablespoons safflower oil
- 1 egg, beaten
- 2 tablespoons honey
- ¼ cup maple syrup

- ½ teaspoon vanilla

- 1 cup Gluten-Free Baking Mix

- 1 teaspoon ground cinnamon

- ¼ teaspoon ground ginger

- ½ cup chopped pecans or walnuts

Instructions

1. Preheat the oven to 350ºF.

2. Grease a 6-cup muffin pan and set it aside.

3. Combine the pumpkin, cran-raspberry sauce, oil, egg, honey, syrup and vanilla in a medium-sized bowl.

4. Combine the remaining ingredients, except for the nuts, and stir this flour mixture into the pumpkin mixture.

5. Stir in the nuts.

6. Fill each muffin cup with a scant 1/2 cup of batter.

7. Bake in the preheated oven for 25-30 minutes, or until a toothpick inserted in the center of a muffin comes out clean.

Pecan Cherry Cookies

Looking for a delicious cookie that is good for you too? These Pecan Cherry cookies are just that. There are only a few ingredients but each one provides you with an abundance of nutrients.

Serves: 9

Ingredients

- 1 cup raw pecans

- ¼ cup unsweetened coconut, shredded

- 2 tablespoons coconut nectar

- 1 tablespoon extra virgin coconut oil

- ⅓ cup unsweetened dried cherries

- 1 teaspoon vanilla

- a pinch of celtic sea salt

Instructions

1. Preheat the over to 350°F

2. Place all of the ingredients into a bowl of a food processor. Process about 20 seconds or until the mixture resembles a fine granola.

3. Divide the dough into 9 portions. Form each into a ball.

4. Place the cookies on baking sheet and lightly press down to flatten.

5. Bake for 8-10 minutes or until the edges just begin to brown. Do not over bake.

Maple Walnut Shortbread Cookies

These Maple Walnut Shortbread cookies, sweetened with maple syrup instead of white sugar and made with ground walnuts and gluten-free flours, taste every bit as buttery and decadent as standard shortbread cookies.

Serves: 12

Ingredients

- ½ cup butter, at room temperature
- 2 tablespoons maple syrup
- 1 teaspoon vanilla
- ¼ cup very finely chopped walnuts
- ¼ cup oat flour

- 2 tablespoons sorghum flour

- 2 tablespoons tapioca flour

- 3 tablespoons potato starch (not potato flour)

- ¼ teaspoon xanthan gum

- ⅛ teaspoon sea salt

Instructions

1. Combine the butter, syrup and vanilla in a mixing bowl. Using an electric mixer, mix on High for 2 minutes.

2. Place the remaining ingredients in a covered container and shake well to ensure ingredients are mixed thoroughly.

3. Add the dry mixture to the mixing bowl and
    mix on Low until combined, about 1 minute.

4. Using a rubber spatula, mix well to ensure
    that all the ingredients are thoroughly
    combined.

5. Spoon the dough onto a sheet of parchment
    paper, making a straight line of dough about
    8 inches long.

6. Fold the paper over the dough and form into
    an 8-inch long by 2-inch wide log.

7. Refrigerate the dough log for about 30
    minutes, or until firm.

8. Slice the log into ½-inch slices and place
    them on a large cookie sheet, leaving 1 inch
    of space around each cookie.

9. Refrigerate the cookies for at least 30 minutes.

10. Preheat the oven to 350ºF.

11. Bake the cookies in the preheated oven for 13-15 minutes, or until the edges begin to brown.

12. Allow the cookies to cool for a few minutes on the baking sheet, and then transfer them to a cooling rack to cool completely.

13. Store the cookies in a tin or cookie jar.